Contents

Picky Eater

Having picky eaters is common. But that doesn't make it any easier! Fortunately, there are ways you can help your kids accept a wider variety of foods and feel more positive during mealtimes. Read on to learn step-by-step strategies for overcoming picky eating, what habits to avoid, and when to call in professional help.

You've just set the table for dinner. It's a simple meal of baked chicken, steamed veggies, and rolls. But before you can even sit down, one of your kids is crying. What's going on?

Your picky eater is upset. And you're not exactly surprised. She doesn't see the food she likes to eat best, and she's melting down.

So what do you do? You watch her sniffle and only eat the rolls. Or you cave and play the short-order cook, getting her a preferred food while the rest of the family eats the main meal.

Neither of these outcomes feels satisfying to anyone. And it's likely to repeat tomorrow. But rest assured, you CAN move the needle on picky eating. We have some strategies that can help.

The first step is to step into your kids' shoes for a minute...

What Your Picky Eater Might Be Feeling

We're often so rooted in our perspective as parents that we can forget that picky eating is hard on our kids, too. But the better we can understand what they're thinking and feeling, the better we can problem-solve and overcome picky eating as a family. Your picky eater might be thinking...

• I don't like the way that food tastes or feels in my mouth.

• I don't feel safe or comforted by this food.

• I've never seen this food before and I have no idea what to expect.

• This food looks like something else I know I don't like.

• I'm worried there's nothing here that I can eat, and I'll go hungry.

• I'm embarrassed or ashamed that I can't face the foods that others are eating.

Picky Eater Progress Plan, Step-by-Step

This plan can help you and your picky eater make incremental steps toward greater food acceptance skills. This kind of plan is often used to help coach kids' with medically-significant feeding challenges to become more accepting of new foods. So it can really work! Try it at home. And as you move through this steps, remember the power of modeling eating well for your kids.

1. Plan family meal time. Eat meals at the table as a family. Do not offer food while your child is playing, watching television or walking around.

2. Be a role model. Your child will eat better and be more willing to try new foods if she sees others at the table eating the same foods. Family members, including older brothers and sisters, are important role models for healthy eating.

3. Eat at regular times. Offer three meals and up to three snacks at regular times each day. Offer only water between meals and snacks. This will keep your child hydrated and will also make sure that she doesn't fill up before meal time. This way she will come to the table hungry.

What if my child won't eat? If your child refuses to eat at snack or mealtime, offer food only at the next scheduled time. Stick to this rule even when your child refuses dinner and has to wait until breakfast. If children eat less at one meal, they will make up for it and eat more at the next meal.

4. Promote happy meal times. Your child will eat better if she is enjoying mealtime. Children are more likely to have a happy meal time if you don't pressure them to eat.

5. Avoid distractions. Meals and snacks should be served away from distractions like the television or computer. Mealtime is for eating and interacting with the family. Do not have toys at the table or on your child's tray. Leave toys, books, television and music for playtime before or after meals.

6. Prepare one meal for the family. Make sure you offer food in the correct texture and size of pieces for your child. Remember it is the parent or caregiver's job to offer the food and it is your child's decision whether they will eat or not. Your child will be more willing to try new foods if she knows she will not get her favourite foods when she refuses dinner.

7. Listen to your child. Trust that your child knows when she is hungry and full.

8. Don't pressure, praise, reward, trick or punish. Children who want to be independent will not eat well if they feel pressure. Allow your

child to decide if or how much she will eat from the foods offered. Trust that she will eat if she is hungry.

9. Try, try again. Continue offering new foods even if your child has said no to them before. Offer these foods on different days, at different meals and in different recipes. It can take as many as 10 times for a child to try a food and like it. Don't give up!

10. Limit meal time. Allow your child a maximum of 30 minutes to eat the meal. After this time put the food away and let your child leave the table. Offer food again at the next scheduled meal or snack time. Extending meal time too

long will not make your child more likely to eat and does not create a healthy and happy eating environment.

Avoid Habits That Can Worsen Picky Eating

Sometimes our best efforts to manage picky eating can actually do more harm than good. Look out for these feeding pitfalls that can prolong picky eating and make it more deeply ingrained. (Don't feel guilty if some of these apply to you!)

• Making separate meals for your picky eater.

• Pressuring your child to eat during meals (this can sound like "just one more bite.")

- Letting your child snacks continuously throughout the day, "grazing" on preferred foods instead of sitting down for planned meals.

- Serving the same foods many days in a row.

- Serving ONLY new foods at dinner, without a balance of "safe" or preferred foods.

- Letting kids decide what's for dinner.

Seek Help for Extreme Picky Eating

If you're concerned that your child's picky eating is more than just a phase, or that it's negatively impacting their nutritional status, it's perfectly OK to seek help from your child's pediatrician. She'll be able to refer you to a feeding expert who can work with you and your child to help customize a program for overcoming these challenges as a family.

Progress Takes Time

The good news is, most kids do grow out of their pickiest phase. Becoming an adventurous eater is a multi-year process, even for "good" eaters. (Are there any foods you didn't learn to like until you were a full-grown adult? Then you know it can really take time!)

As we tell our kids, we have to "practice our patience." Keep offering a variety of healthy foods, some new and some familiar, and enjoy the journey as much as you're able.

Picky Eating: 10 Fun Tips to Get Kids to Try New Foods

Does your child say no to new foods? Getting your child to try something new can be frustrating. It can make mealtimes stressful for you, your child and the rest of the family. Try these ideas to get your child more interested in trying new foods.

1. Get your kids involved in the kitchen. Children can wash fruit and vegetables, tear lettuce, mix batter or push the buttons on the microwave. Help your child if he is too young to do these tasks on his own.

2. Work together. Children can set the table and take the family's drink "orders" to help prepare for mealtime. Get the whole family to work together.

3. Try gardening. Plant a garden and watch it grow! Good starter vegetables are carrots, cucumbers, green beans, lettuce, tomatoes, peppers, zucchini, radishes, peas and onions.

4. Plan together. Involve your kids in the meal planning process. Let them help choose a healthy meal once a week. Print this menu planning worksheet to get started.

5. Get creative. Present foods in creative ways. Cut sandwiches into fun shapes with a knife or cookie cutter. Try these fun "foodimals" which are foods shaped like animals!

6. Try kid-approved recipes. Try these healthy and fun kid-approved recipes from our Kids Recipe Challenge.

7. Have a dinner theme night. Choose dishes that come from different parts of the world. Try Mexican, Chinese, African, Caribbean, Indian, Italian, Thai, Eastern European, Middle Eastern, Swedish, Vietnamese or Ethiopian.

8. Learn through games and activities. Play games and do activities to learn about food. Put mystery foods in a paper bag and guess which foods they are by feeling or smelling them. Get your child to draw her own place mat with her favourite foods or solve funny riddles. Here's a fun colouring activity to try.

9. Go on a field trip! Take an adventure to the pumpkin patch, a corn maze or your local farmers market. Even a grocery store in a different neighbourhood might have new vegetables and fruit to learn about. See what your family can discover!

10. Make it fun! Have nights where you have breakfast for dinner; make your own pizza night; build your own yogurt sundae bar; or just snack on veggies and dip with popcorn for dessert.

Why Are Some Kids Pickier About Food Than Others?

Many different factors can impact a child's willingness to taste new foods and yes, some kids won't even come near a new food, much less touch it! When I assess a child to determine why they have difficulty eating a variety of foods, I look closely at three factors: First, the child's physiology.

While typically gastrointestinal in nature, it may also be something as simple as a cavity, which the child then associated with crunchy foods, and begins to only eat soft foods.

It takes a bit of detective work! Included in the category of physiology is the sensory system and how the child is able to take in information through his senses and respond appropriately. For example, the texture of Stage 3 baby foods may provide too much sensory input for some babies, yet the smoother textures in the earlier stages were never a problem.

Second, I look closely at the child's oral motor skills. Does he have the strength and stability in the oral structures to learn to chew more advanced foods? If not, he may stall at the "soft table foods" stage and appear picky when parents offer more advanced foods that require more chewing. He quickly learns that he cannot eat the more challenging textures and refuses them.

Third, I observe and identify the behaviors that he has learned in order to avoid eating. This includes behavior around food and family dynamics in general. Discovering why a child is a picky eater takes time and helping him to become a more adventurous eater requires patience and yes, more time!

Tips for How Parents Can Avoid Power Struggles With a Picky Eater

Resist the urge to say "See, I told you that you would like it!" after a child finally gives in and takes a bite. Well-meaning parents believe they are being supportive and don't realize that it's patronizing and not a helpful comment.

Instead, let the child make the decision to taste it at their own pace and pause, letting them tell you how they felt about it. If they don't like the taste, you can praise them for trying it by saying "Wow, you are very brave! It's not easy to try new things, but you did it!" or "I bet your taste buds are wondering what the next new food will be…you're teaching your tongue about new foods! What a terrific teacher you are!"

Catch your child being good to his body. If you notice him requesting an apple, use that as a teaching moment. Perhaps you might talk about why apples are good for our bodies or you might say "You know, when I was a little boy, I didn't like apples. How did you learn to be such an amazing apple eater? I'm going to try more apples, just like you."

Raising an adventurous eater means raising a child who makes healthy decisions about what goes into his body and what fuels him best for his day. When children begin to make their own informed decisions (with our guidance, much like authoritative parenting) about how much they eat and which foods feel good in their bodies, it eliminates the power struggle and provides a healthier atmosphere in the family home.

Picky Eaters: Commonly Asked Questions

Children sometimes don't eat as well as you would like. Some children have a short list of foods they will eat and others simply refuse to try new foods. Read on for quick answers to some common questions about feeding picky eaters.

How can I get my child to try new foods?

Children need to see a new food many times before they will actually eat it. Try these tips:

• Put a new food on your child's plate for him to look at and experiment with. Have him try "one bite". This can help increase comfort and acceptance of new foods.

• Build up your child's list of acceptable foods by adding a few new foods each day or week. For example, if she always wants a cheese sandwich for lunch, change the vegetables, fruit or soups you serve with it.

• Avoid force feeding or offering a reward for tasting new foods as this may decrease acceptance.

• Be a good role model! Eating with parents, siblings or peers who are enjoying new foods can help.

• Involve your child in making a meal. Children who help make a meal are more likely to eat it!

My child snacks all day and then won't eat supper – what can I do?

Children can fill up easily if they snack all day.

• Offer healthy snacks at least one to two hours before meals. Closer to meal times, offer a plate of cut up fruit or raw vegetable sticks.

• Avoid high fat chips, cookies or other baked goods as snacks since they are low in nutrients and very filling.

• Get your child to be active throughout the day to build his appetite.

My child eats a lot of bread and cereal. Is that okay?

The amount of grain products like bread and cereal that children need depends on their age. Watch this video to find out how many servings your child needs. When choosing breads and cereals, try these tips.

• Look for whole grain breads and cereals made with 100% whole grain whole wheat, oatmeal, rye, pumpernickel, barley or corn.

• Use the nutrition facts label to help you choose breads and cereals that are higher in fibre and lower in sugar.

• Offer other foods with breads like egg, hummus or cut up chicken.

• Offer other foods with cereals like cut up fruit and yogurt.

What can I do if my child won't eat meat?

Avoiding meat is not a concern as long as your child is getting the nutrients she needs from other foods. Foods such as eggs, beans, peas, lentils, nuts, seeds, tofu and fortified meat alternatives like veggie burgers can take the place of meat. Try these tips:

• Make an egg salad with 2 eggs, a creamy dressing, celery and cucumbers

• Add beans to your favourite chili recipe

• Add tofu to a vegetable stir fry

• Spread peanut butter on whole grain crackers with apple slices on the side

• Sprinkle a combination of walnuts, almonds and flaxseeds on a yogurt smoothie

• Try carrot sticks dipped hummus

Cooking with Kids of Different Ages

Cooking food together with kids lets you share food and cooking traditions and important food skills. If your kids get cooking now, chances are they will keep up this good habit as they grow older.

Read on for tips to get your kids cooking and get great recipes to try. Cooking with your:

- 2-3 year old

- 3-4 year old

- 4-6 year old

- 6-8 year old

- 8-11 year old

Cooking with 2-3 year olds

Very young children like to explore with their senses of sight, touch, smell, hearing and tasting. They also like to do things on their own. Try letting your kids:

• Wash fruits and vegetables in the sink

• Add items to dishes (like chopped tofu to a casserole)

• Smell food, herbs and spices you are using

• Help find ingredients in the fridge or cupboard

• Put paper cups into muffin tins

Keep in mind, some kids may be happy to watch you cook and talk about what you are doing. An empty pot on the floor with a spoon keeps their hands busy. Be sure to ask lots of questions about what they are making that smells so good!

Cooking with 3-4 year olds

At this age, children may be more interested in talking than eating! Either way, cooking keeps them interested in food. Try letting your kids:

• Remove eggshells from hard-boiled eggs

• Pour from a small pitcher or measuring cup

• Make a simple sandwich or pizza with pre-assembled ingredients

• Describe the colour, taste and shape of food

• Mash sweet potatoes, turnips, carrots or bananas

Cooking with 4-6 year olds

At this age, some kids may show signs of being a picky eater. While the food they prepare might not make it to their fork, try to be patient knowing that cooking is helping them warm up to the idea of trying new foods. Try letting your kids:

• Assemble foods: make trail mix or their own yogurt smoothie with toppings you've prepared

• Stir ingredients together (like muffins, pancakes, sauces)

• Slice soft-cooked vegetables, soft fruit, cheese or tofu with a plastic knife

• Crack and beat an egg

• Cook with a friend for a fun play date

Cooking with 6-8 year olds

At this age, kids can follow simple steps for recipes and are able to share and take turns. Try letting your kids:

- Use simple kitchen equipment such as a grater, toaster, blender or can opener after you show them how to do so safely

- Make simple cold spring rolls or tortilla wraps

- Toss salad ingredients together with salad dressing

- Invent a fruit salad or smoothie recipe

- Write a list of healthy snacks they like to eat

- Write out a grocery list

- Make a simple breakfast: whole grain cereal with milk or canned fruit over yogurt

Cooking with 8-11 year olds

Kids at this age are more coordinated and able to understand how to use appliances safely. Try letting your kids:

- Use a knife with easy-to-cut foods (cooked meats, cheese, tofu, breads)

- Use the microwave with your help

- Make their own school lunch

- Make a fresh fruit platter to go with dinner

- Use the stove, with supervision, to make basic recipes: omelets, pancakes, quesadillas, soups or grilled cheese

- Decide what is needed to balance out a meal so it has food from each food group

Kid friendly award winning recipes

Kid friendly award winning recipes

- Coconut Cashew Curry Chicken

This spiced up chicken is saucy enough to serve over rice alongside your favourite vegetables.

- Colourful Layered Sandwich

This colourful sandwich can be changed for each lunch depending on what you have available in your fridge and pantry and what your kids enjoy eating.

- Creamy Zucchini Dip

This vegetable dip is perfect to serve up with crunchy vegetables.

- Crispy Kale Chips

Kale chips are a fun way to enjoy this tasty green. Change up the flavours and get creative with spices!

- Crunchy Peanut Butter Boat

This recipe comes to us from Jasmin in North Bay, who shared this twist on a banana and peanut butter favourite.

- Souper Lunch with Rice and Beans

Full of vegetables and flavour, this soup will keep warm tucked in a thermos for lunch on a cold winter day.

- Soy Butter and Banana Roll

Your kids will love this twist on the traditional peanut butter and banana sandwich.

- Spicy Grilled Cheese

Kids of all ages love grilled cheese sandwiches for lunch.

- Spicy Turkey Vegetable Casserole

All-in-one casseroles always make dinner easy.

- Stephen's Curried Eggs

This recipe will be a favourite for kids that love flavours and experiencing new tastes.

- Green Meatballs

Jillian's recipe inspired this green meatball version to enjoy hot from a thermos or cold packed in kids' lunches

- Ground up Frog Smoothie

This is a smoothie that will appeal to a kids' sense of humour and taste buds

- Hawaiian Enchiladas

This recipe is a spin on a pizza favourite! Use different toppings to change up the flavours.

- Hearty Chicken and Vegetable Salad

This salad packs a protein punch and is filled with a variety of vegetables that kids can help prepare.

- Hungry Kids Sundae

This fun fruit filled snack plays on the "sundae" theme with a healthy twist. Cut the fruit and prepare the ingredients and then let kids play with this healthy sundae bar.

BABY & TOT PICKY EATER MEAL PLAN

It seems we constantly hear about kids being picky eaters; it may feel like we are condemned to have a child who will eat nothing but chicken fingers and pizza. Is there anything you can do to raise an adventurous eater? Plenty actually, starting right now!

Family meals are one of the best ways to encourage an adventurous eater. Family meals promote better nutrition, eating habits and even behavior.

Babies and toddlers learn to eat from you! Babies and tots are more likely to try foods they see their parents eat. Make sure you are modeling good eating behavior. In one survey of parents of preschool age children, the parents' fruit and vegetable consumption was the strongest predictor of how much of these foods the kids ate.

Little ones tend to like new foods paired with an existing favorite. Try to use your child's favorite foods to add new ones.

Meal and snack schedules are very important so babies and toddlers arrive to the table hungry and wanting to eat. Don't let snacks get within 1-1.5 hours of a meal.

It's also important to practice what's known as the "division of responsibility". As the caregiver, you provide the time, place, and choices for eating. Your child decides whether to eat and how much to eat.

Pro-tip:

If your child doesn't seem to like a new food, don't pay too much attention. He may need many exposures to foods before he readily accepts them. Be patient and try cooking foods differently (sautéed, roasted, steamed) or with different flavors to help baby learn to like them. It might take up to 10-20 times before they like it! Avoid pressuring your child to eat a food. This can backfire. Instead, use the "parent provides, child decides" philosophy – parents choose which foods are offered, but your baby should be allowed to choose whether to eat, which foods to choose and how much to eat.

The below meals and snacks provide a variety of flavors and textures to help raise an adventurous eater!

Breakfast

- Option 1: Whole grain toast topped with nut butter and sliced bananas

- Option 2: Yogurt Recipe: Berry Muesli

- Option 3: Omelet with finely diced bell pepper and mushrooms

- Option 4: Whole grain waffle with ricotta cheese and berries

- Option 5: Yogurt and quinoa parfait with cinnamon pears

Lunch

- Option 1: Yogurt Recipe: Cheesy Peasy Pasta

- Option 2: Turkey roll up-whole wheat tortilla with hummus spread, turkey and sliced cucumber

- Option 3: Quesadilla made with whole-wheat tortillas, cheddar cheese and cubed avocado

- Option 4: Whole grain toast with light tuna and carrots

- Option 5: Tex-Mex pizza: whole grain pita topped with tomato sauce, cheddar cheese, and black or pinto beans

Dinner

- Option 1: Whole grain spaghetti with tomato sauce and ground beef, chicken or turkey mixed with soft cooked mushrooms

- Option 2: Baked fish with green beans and a sweet potato

- Option 3: Cheeseburger (ground beef, chicken or turkey), cut up in pieces on a whole grain roll and soft roasted zucchini

- Option 4: Stir fry with chicken, squash, peas and brown rice

- Option 5: Breaded baked chicken strips with steamed carrots and a whole grain dinner roll

Snacks

- Option 1: Yogurt Recipe: Sweet Yogurt Dip

- Option 2: Cottage cheese and fruit

- Option 3: Veggies with hummus dip

- Option 4: Yogurt Recipe: Fruit & Yogurt Pops

- Option 5: Yogurt Recipe: Blueberry Banana Blender Muffins

PICKY EATERS DIET RECIPES

In this part are picky eaters diet recipes delicious recipes every picky eaters would love

Cheesy American Goulash

Preparation time

Ingredients

- 1 tablespoon olive oil

- 1 medium onion, diced

- 1 teaspoon paprika

- 1 teaspoon Italian seasoning

- ½ teaspoon salt

- ½ teaspoon black pepper

- 1 lb ground beef

- 2 cloves garlic, minced

- 15 ounce can crushed tomatoes

- 15 ounce can fire roasted diced tomatoes

- 1 cup water

- 1 cup dry elbow macaroni

- 1 cup shredded Cheddar cheese

Instructions

1. Preheat oven to 400F.

2. In a large, oven proof skillet, heat oil over medium-high heat. Add the onions, sauté until soft, about 2 to 3 minutes. Add the paprika, Italian seasoning, salt, and black pepper, sauté for an additional minute.

3. Add the ground beef, breaking up the meat with a wooden spoon or spatula, as it cooks. Cook for 7 minutes.

4. Stir in the garlic, crushed tomatoes, diced tomatoes (including the liquid), and water. Bring to a simmer.

5. Add the pasta to the goulash. Cover and transfer the skillet to the preheated oven. Bake for 22 to 25 minutes or until the pasta is tender and sauce thickened. Top with cheese and return

to the oven, uncovered, until the cheese is melted.

Chicken Zucchini Casserole

Preparation time

55 minutes

Ingredients

- 6 ounces boxed stuffing mix (such as Stove Top)

- ½ cup butter melted

- 4 zucchini diced

- 3 boneless, skinless chicken breasts cooked and diced

- 10 ½ ounces canned cream of chicken soup

- ½ onion diced

- ½ cup sour cream

Instructions

1. Preheat oven to 350 degrees F.

2. In a large bowl, combine the stuffing mix and melted butter. Set aside 1/2 cup of the mixture for topping.

3. Add zucchini, cooked chicken, cream of chicken soup, onion and sour cream to the stuffing in the large bowl.

4. Spread zucchini mixture in an even layer in a 9 x 13 inch glass pan sprayed with nonstick cooking spray.

5. Sprinkle reserved stuffing mix on top and bake, uncovered, for 40-50 minutes or until cooked through and the top is golden brown.

PEACH COBBLER DUMP CAKE

Preparation time

50 minutes

Ingredients

- 2 (16 ounce) cans peaches in heavy syrup (undrained)

- 1 (15.25 ounce) package yellow cake mix

- 1/2 cup butter

- 1/2 teaspoon ground cinnamon

- 1 quart vanilla ice cream - optional topping

Instructions

1. Preheat oven to 375 degrees F.

2. Empty peaches into the bottom of a 9 x 13 inch baking pan.

3. Cover with the dry cake mix and press down firmly.

4. Cut butter into small pieces and place on top of cake mix.

5. Sprinkle top with cinnamon.

6. Bake for 45 minutes.

7. Serve with vanilla ice cream, if desired.

Creamy Pumpkin Pasta with Pine Nut Gremolata

Preparation time

25 minutes

INGREDIENTS

- 12 oz. rigatoni

- 2 tbsp. olive oil, divided

- 12 fresh sage leaves

- 1/4 c. pine nuts, toasted and roughly chopped

- 1 tsp. finely grated lemon zest

- 1 shallot, finely chopped

- 2 cloves garlic, pressed

- Kosher salt and freshly ground black pepper

- 1 c. canned pure pumpkin

- 2 oz. Parmesan cheese, grated (about 1/2 cup), plus more for serving

- 1/4 c. heavy cream

- 1/8 tsp. fresh grated nutmeg

Instructions

1. Cook pasta per package directions.

2. Reserve 1 cup cooking water; drain pasta and return to pot.

3. Heat 1 tablespoon oil in a large saucepan over medium heat. Add sage and cook until crisp, 2 to 3 minutes.

4. Transfer with a slotted spoon to a paper towel-lined plate; when cool, crumble into pieces.

5. Toss together sage, pine nuts, and lemon zest in a bowl.

6. Add remaining 1 tablespoon oil, shallot, and garlic to saucepan. Season with salt and pepper.

7. Cook, stirring occasionally, until tender, 1 to 2 minutes. Add pumpkin, Parmesan, heavy cream, nutmeg, and 1/2 cup reserved pasta water. Cook until slightly thickened, 3 to 5 minutes.

8.   Season with salt. (If desired, use an immersion blender or standard blender to puree until smooth.)

9.   Add pasta and stir to combine (add more pasta water if sauce seems too thick).

10. Serve sprinkled with Pine Nut Gremolata.

Grilled Hot Dogs with Fixin's

Preparation time

30 minutes

INGREDIENTS

• Grilled Hot Dogs

• 8 hot dogs

- 1 package hot dog buns

Zesty Pickle and Onion Fixin'

- 4 finely chopped pickles

- 1/4 finely chopped small white onion

- 3 tbsp. fresh flat-leaf parsley

- 2 tbsp. whole-grain mustard

- Kosher salt

- Black pepper

Tangy Horseradish Fixin'

- 3 tbsp. prepared horseradish

- 2 tbsp. sour cream

- 1 tbsp. white wine vinegar

- 1 tbsp. mayonnaise

- 1 tsp. sugar

- 1/4 head finely shredded purple cabbage (about 2 cups)

- 1 finely copped scallion

- 1 grated large carrot

- 2 tbsp. chopped fresh dill

- Kosher salt

- Black pepper

Spicy Chiles Fixin'

- 1 c. white wine vinegar

- 2 tbsp. sugar

- 1 tsp. coriander seeds

- 1/4 tsp. kosher salt

- 2 thinly sliced Fresno chiles

- 1 thinly sliced medium red onion

Instructions

1. Grill 8 hot dogs over medium-high heat, turning often, until slightly charred and heated through, 4 to 5 minutes.

2. If desired, grill the buns until lightly toasted.

3. Serve with any or all of the following fixin's.

Make Zesty Pickle and Onion Fixin':

1. Stir together pickles, white onion, fresh flat-leaf parsley, and whole-grain mustard in a bowl.

2. Season with kosher salt and black pepper. Makes about 2 cups.

Make Tangy Horseradish Fixin':

1. Whisk together prepared horseradish (squeezed of excess moisture), sour cream, white wine vinegar, mayonnaise, and sugar in a bowl.

2. Add purple cabbage (about 2 cups), scallion, carrot, and fresh dill.

3. Season with kosher salt and pepper.

4. Let sit, tossing occasionally, for 15 minutes. Makes 2 cups.

Make Spicy Chiles Fixin':

1. Bring white wine vinegar, sugar, coriander seeds, and kosher salt to a simmer in a small pot over medium heat.

2. Remove from heat and add Fresno chiles and red onion.

3. Let sit, tossing occasionally, at least 25 minutes or up to 3 days. Makes 1 1/2 cups.

Cauliflower Mac 'n' Cheese

Preparation time

1 hour

INGREDIENTS

• 3 tbsp. olive oil, divided, plus more for baking dish

• 1 lb. cavatappi or other short pasta

• 1 medium-sized head cauliflower (about 2 pounds), cored and thinly sliced

• 4 cloves garlic, sliced

• 1 large yellow onion, thinly sliced

- Kosher salt and freshly ground black pepper

- 4 oz. extra-sharp white Cheddar cheese, grated (about 1 cup)

- 2 oz. Parmesan cheese, grated (about 1/2 cup)

- 1/4 tsp. mustard powder

- Pinch cayenne pepper

- 1 1/2 c. panko breadcrumbs

- 1/2 c. fresh flat-leaf parsley, chopped

Instructions

1. Preheat oven to 425°F.

2. Lightly oil a 9-by-13-inch baking dish.

3. Cook pasta according to package directions. Drain.

4. Heat 2 tablespoons oil in a large pot over medium heat. Add cauliflower, garlic, and onion.

5. Season with salt.

6. Cook, covered, stirring occasionally, until tender, 15 to 20 minutes.

7. Add 4 cups water and simmer until vegetables are very soft, 10 to 12 minutes.

8. Drain, reserving 2 cups cooking liquid; let cool slightly.

9. Combine vegetables, Cheddar, Parmesan, mustard powder, and cayenne in a blender (depending on the size of your blender, you may need to do this in two batches).

10. Purée, adding just enough reserved cooking liquid to get mixture moving, until smooth, 1 to 2 minutes.

11. Add sauce to pasta and toss to combine.

12. Transfer to prepared baking dish.

13.   Toss together panko, parsley, and remaining tablespoon oil in a bowl.

14. Season with salt and pepper. Sprinkle over pasta.

15. Bake until golden brown, 14 to 16 minutes.

Cornflake-Crusted Baked Chicken

Preparation time

1 hour 30 minutes

INGREDIENTS

- 1 tsp. garlic powder

- 2 1/2 c. buttermilk, divided

- 1 tsp. celery seed, divided

- 1/2 tsp. cayenne pepper, plus a pinch, divided

- Kosher salt and freshly ground black pepper

- 4 small chicken drumsticks, skin removed

- 4 small bone-in chicken thighs, skin removed

- 1 c. all-purpose flour

- 4 c. cornflakes cereal, crushed

- Sliced dill pickles, for serving

Instructions

1. Preheat oven to 425°F.

2. Combine garlic powder, 1 1/2 cups buttermilk, and 1/2 teaspoon each celery seed, cayenne, and salt in a bowl.

3. Add chicken and marinate in refrigerator for 30 minutes.

4. Fit a rack over a large rimmed baking sheet lined with heavy-duty foil.

5. Combine flour, pinch of cayenne, and remaining 1/2 teaspoon celery seed in a bowl.

6. Season with salt and pepper.

7. Place remaining 1 cup buttermilk in a second bowl; season with salt and pepper.

8. Place cornflakes in a third bowl.

9. Remove chicken from marinade, letting excess drip off; discard marinade.

10. Coat chicken with flour mixture, dip in buttermilk, then coat with cornflakes, pressing gently to help adhere.

11. Arrange chicken on prepared baking sheet.

12. Bake until cooked through, 25 to 27 minutes.

13. Serve with pickles alongside.

Ground Turkey Sloppy Joes

Preparation time

30 minutes

INGREDIENTS

- 2 tbsp. olive oil

- 1 medium yellow onion, chopped

- 1 red bell pepper, chopped

- 1 carrot, chopped

- Kosher salt and freshly ground black pepper

- 2 cloves garlic, pressed

- 1 lb. lean ground turkey or chicken

- 1 tbsp. chili powder

- 1/4 tsp. ground cinnamon

- 1 (8-ounce) can tomato sauce

- 1/4 c. sweet relish

- 2 tsp. Worcestershire sauce

- 2 tbsp. red wine vinegar, divided

- 3 Persian cucumbers, thinly sliced

- 1/2 c. thinly sliced red onion

- 6 thick slices toast or split burger buns

Instructions

1. Heat oil in a large skillet over medium heat.

2. Add yellow onion, bell pepper, and carrot. Season with salt and pepper.

3. Cook, stirring occasionally, until tender, 6 to 8 minutes. Add garlic and cook, stirring occasionally, until fragrant, 30 seconds.

4. Add turkey and cook, breaking it up with a spoon, until no longer pink, 4 to 6 minutes.

5. Add chili powder and cinnamon.

6. Cook, stirring occasionally, 1 minute.

7. Add tomato sauce and relish.

8. Simmer until beginning to thicken, 2 to 4 minutes.

9. Stir in Worcestershire and 1 tablespoon vinegar.

10. Toss together cucumbers, red onion, and remaining tablespoon vinegar in a bowl.

11. Season with salt. Let sit, tossing occasionally, 4 to 6 minutes.

12. Spoon meat mixture on top of toast and top with pickles.

EASY CLASSIC SHEPHERD'S PIE

Preparation time

1 hour

Ingredients

• 2 pounds ground lamb

• 2 tablespoons of oil

• 1 medium onion chopped

- 2 garlic cloves minced

- 1 15 oz can sliced carrots drained

- 1 15 oz can green beans drained

- 1 4 oz can sliced mushrooms

- 1 tablespoon ketchup

- 2 tablespoons tomato paste

- 1 tablespoon Worcestershire sauce

- 1 teaspoon dried rosemary

- 1 tablespoon garlic powder

- Salt/pepper to taste

- 6 cups prepared instant mashed potatoes

- 3 tablespoons margarine melted

- 3 tablespoons grated Parmesan cheese

Instructions

1. Heat the oven to 375°F.

2. While the oven is heating, add oil to a large skillet over medium to high heat.

3. Add the ground lamb, onion, and garlic to the skillet and cook until the lamb is brown, stirring often to separate meat.

4. Drain off any fat and transfer to a large bowl.

5. Stir in carrots, green beans, mushrooms, ketchup, tomato paste, Worcestershire sauce, rosemary, and garlic powder. Stir until combined and season with salt/pepper to taste.

6. Pour the lamb mixture into a 13×9 inch casserole dish and spoon the mashed potatoes on top.

7. Drizzle the melted margarine and Parmesan cheese on top and bake for about 40 minutes or until the topping is lightly browned.

8. Enjoy!

MISSISSIPPI POT ROAST (NO PEPPERONCINI)

Preparation time

8 hours 15 minutes

ingredients

- 2 tablespoons cooking oil

- 4 pound chuck roast

- 2 tablespoons Soul Dust, or another salt, pepper, and garlic blend

- 2 tablespoons Sweet Heat, or another type of all purpose seasoning such as Lawry's

- 1/4 cup all purpose flour

- 1/2 cup unsalted butter

- 1 packet of Au Jus

- 1 packed of Ranch seasoning

- mashed potatoes, for serving

Instructions

1. Preheat cooking oil in skillet over medium high heat.

2. Season chuck roast with Soul Dust (or a salt, pepper, and garlic mixture) and Sweet Heat (or another type of all purpose seasoning like Lawry's).

3. Add 1/4 cup flour to a plate or shallow bowl.

4. Coat all sides of chuck roast in flour.

5. Add roast to hot skillet and brown on all sides. About 3-4 minutes per side.

6. Add roast to slow cooker.

7. Add butter and sprinkle Au Jus and Ranch seasoning to slow cooker.

8. Cook on Low Heat for 8 hours until meat is fork tender.

9. Serve over mashed potatoes.

PHILLY CHEESESTEAK PASTA

Preparation time

20 minutes

INGREDIENTS

For the Pasta:

- 10 ounces cavatappi pasta

- Fine sea salt and freshly cracked pepper

For the Veggies

- 2 tablespoons unsalted butter

- 1 cup thinly-sliced yellow onion

- 1 and 1/2 cups thinly-sliced green pepper

- 1 cup (3.5 ounces) sliced mushrooms,

- 1 teaspoon minced garlic

- 1 tablespoon red wine vinegar

For the Beef:

- 1 pound lean ground beef

- 1 tbsp Italian seasoning

- For the Provolone Sauce:

- 4 tablespoons unsalted butter

- 4 tablespoons all-purpose flour

- 1 cup whole milk

* 1 cup low sodium beef stock

* 1 and 1/2 cups shredded Italian cheese blend

Optional:

* 4 slices provolone cheese

* Fresh chopped parsley for garnish

* Get IngredientsPowered by Chicory

INSTRUCTIONS

For the Pasta:

1. Fill a large pot with water and bring it to a boil.

2. Add a pinch of salt to the water, followed by the pasta.

3. Cook the pasta according to package instructions or until al dente. Strain the pasta through a colander and set aside.

For the Veggies

1. In a large OVEN SAFE skillet (that will fit everything for the final dish) over medium-high heat, add the butter.

2. Next, add the thinly sliced onion, green pepper, and mushrooms.

3. Add a tiny pinch salt and pepper to taste.

4. Saute the veggies until they are softened and golden brown, about 10 minutes. (If you need to add a little water to the pan to prevent the veggies from sticking that's okay!) In the last 30

seconds of cooking, add the garlic and cook until fragrant.

5. Remove the skillet from the heat and stir in the red wine vinegar.

6. Pour the peppers and onions into the colander with the pasta.

For the Beef:

1. Preheat the oven to a HIGH broil. In the same skillet, add the ground beef and Italian seasoning.

2. Crumble the beef as you cook until it is completely browned through.

3. Drain off any fat.

4. Add the pasta and veggies from the colandar into the skillet with the beef.

For the Provolone Sauce:

1. In the same pot you used to cook the pasta in, add the butter and heat to medium heat.

2. Let the butter melt and then whisk in the flour. Keep whisking for a minute or until you cook out all of the raw flour taste.

3. Gradually add the milk and beef stock.

4. Stir often so the mixture doesn't clump.

5. After about 5 minutes the sauce should thicken, then add the shredded Italian cheese blend. Stir until melted and smooth.

6.   Turn off the heat and pour the sauce over skillet with the beef, peppers, onions and pasta.

7. Toss to make sure everything is well combined. Taste and season with salt and pepper as needed (might not need any).

8. You can eat the dish at this point OR add more cheese.

9. Place the slices of provolone on top of the oven safe skillet and broil for 1-2 minutes in the oven or until cheese is nice and melty.

10. Remove and serve, garnish if desired with fresh chopped parsley.

HOT DOG NUGGETS

Preparation time

18 minutes

Ingredients

• 5 hot dogs

• 1 can crescent rolls

• ketchup and mustard for dipping

Instructions

1. Begin by preheating you oven to 400 degrees.

2. Slice your hot dogs into thin pieces (ours were about half inch each). Set aside.

3. Roll out your crescent dough and press the seams together.

4. Cut into 8 strips.

5. Then cut lengthwise into 8 more strips. You should end up with 64 1.5 inch x .5 inch pieces.

6. Wrap the hot dogs in the crescent pieces and place on a parchment paper lined baking sheet.

7. Bake for 8 to 9 minutes. Serve warm. ENJOY!

Cheesy Chicken Broccoli Rice Casserole

Preparation time

1 hour

Ingredients

- 1 (6 oz) package long-grain and wild rice mix

- 3 tablespoons unsalted butter

- 3 cloves garlic minced

- 1 onion diced

- 2 cups cremini mushrooms quartered

- 1 stalk celery diced

- 1/2 teaspoon dried thyme

- 1 tablespoon all-purpose flour

- 1/4 cup dry white wine

- 1 1/2 cups chicken broth

- Kosher salt and freshly ground black pepper to taste

- 3 cups broccoli florets

- 1/2 cup sour cream

- 2 cups shredded rotisserie chicken

- 1 cup shredded cheddar cheese divided (can use reduced fat)

- 2 tablespoons chopped fresh parsley leaves for garnish, optional

Instructions

1. Preheat oven to 375 degrees F.

2. Cook the rice mix according to package instructions; set aside.

3. Melt the butter in a large ovenproof skillet over medium-high heat.

4. Add the garlic, onion, mushrooms, and celery and cook, stirring occasionally, until tender, 3 to 4 minutes.

5. Stir in the thyme and cook until fragrant, about 1 minute.

6. Whisk in the flour until lightly browned, about 1 minute.

7. Gradually whisk in the wine and chicken broth.

8. Cook, whisking constantly, until slightly thickened, 2 to 3 minutes; season with salt and pepper to taste.

9. Stir in the broccoli, sour cream, chicken, ½ cup of the cheese, and the rice.

10. If you want to freeze the casserole, you can stop here and skip to step 7.

11. Otherwise, sprinkle with the remaining ½ cup cheese.

12. Transfer the skillet to the oven and bake until the casserole is bubbly and heated through, 20 to 22 minutes.

13. Serve immediately, garnish with parsley, if desired.

Note

1. To freeze, transfer the unbaked casserole mixture to a ziplock freezer bag and lay the bag flat in the freezer.

2. Freeze for up to 3 months.

3. When ready to serve, thaw overnight in the refrigerator.

4. To cook, transfer to an ovenproof skillet or baking pan, sprinkle with ½ cup cheddar cheese, and bake at 375 degrees F for 20 to 30 minutes, or until heated through.

CREAMY PUMPKIN PASTA WITH TOASTED WALNUTS AND SPINACH

Preparation time

15 minutes

Ingredients

- 8 ounces shells or bowtie pasta

- 1 tbsp Extra Virgin Olive Oil

- 2 cloves fresh garlic, minced

- 1 cup pure pumpkin puree (I used canned)

- 2 tbsp tomato paste

- 2 tbsp half and half (Swap in coconut milk for a vegan sauce.)

- 1 cup vegetable broth

- pinch ground nutmeg

- Cracked black pepper and salt to taste

- 2 cups baby spinach, heaping

- 1/4 cup chopped toasted walnuts

- Parmesan cheese (Optional; Use crushed walnuts for a vegan recipe.)

Instructions

1. Cook the pasta according to package instructions. Drain and set aside but keep it warm.

2. While the pasta cooks, bring a large skillet to medium heat and add the olive oil and minced garlic.

3. Cook just until fragrant.

4. Whisk in the tomato paste, pumpkin, half and half until smooth.

5. Add the vegetable broth, nutmeg, salt and pepper.

6. Stir until combined. Let cook on low about 5 minutes.

7. Add the spinach.

8. Cook until it lightly wilts.

9. Stir in pasta and toss to coat.

10. Sprinkle with walnuts and Parmesan, if desired and serve.

Easy Meatball Subs

Preparation time

35 minutes

Ingredients

- 1 tablespoon plus 1 teaspoon olive oil

- 2 medium garlic cloves, pressed

- 2 teaspoons dried oregano

- 1 pinch red pepper flakes, (big or small pinch, depending on how much heat your crowd likes)

- 1 28-ounce can crushed tomatoes

- 1/2 teaspoon salt

- 1/2 teaspoon sugar

- 1 package Rosina Italian Style Meatballs, (1/2 ounce size)

- 6 sub, brat, or hot dog buns

- 3/4 cup shredded mozzarella cheese

Instructions

- In a medium skillet or saucepan, heat olive oil on medium heat for 15 seconds, then add garlic, oregano, and red pepper flakes and cook, stirring constantly, for 1 minute.

- Add crushed tomatoes and stir well; add salt and sugar and stir again until combined

- Add entire package of Rosina Italian Style Meatballs to sauce, stirring so meatballs are covered in sauce.

- Cover pan and cook for 20-25 minutes, stirring occasionally.

- Move oven rack to top position, and heat the broiler to HIGH.

- Spoon saucy meatballs into buns, top with cheese, and place on a baking sheet under the broiler for 1-2 minutes, checking frequently to make sure they don't burn.

Pizza Quesadillas

Preparation time

11 minutes

Ingredients

- 1 tortilla

- 2 Tablespoons marinara or pizza sauce

- ¼ c. shredded mozzarella cheese

- Optional additional ingredients: grated Parmesan cheese, sliced pepperoni, mushrooms, onions, bell peppers, sausage, or any other pizza toppings of your choice

- For dipping: warm marinara sauce

Instructions

1. Preheat a flat griddle or a large skillet over medium heat.

2. Spread marinara sauce on half of the tortilla.

3. Sprinkle with shredded mozzarella cheese, and any other toppings of your choice.

4. Add another layer of mozzarella over toppings.

5. Fold tortilla over.

6. Spray griddle with cooking spray and cook quesadilla for 2-3 minutes per side, or until browned.

7. Remove to a cutting board and allow the quesadilla to cool for a few minutes. Cut into triangles and serve.

Instant Pot Southern Macaroni and Cheese

Preparation time

40 minutes

Ingredients

• 1 Cup Mozzarella Cheese Farm Style Cut Tillamook, Shredded

• 1 Cup Cheddar Cheese Tillamook Sharp, Loaf

- 1 Cup Cheddar Cheese Tillamook Special Reserve Extra Sharp Loaf

- 1 Ounce Cream Cheese softened

- Dash Hot Sauce

- Dash Nutmeg

- 1 Teaspoon Mustard Ground Dry

- 1/4-1/2 Teaspoon Salt to taste

- 14.5 Ounces Chicken Stock

- 2 Cups Water

- 1 1/2 Tablespoons Butter Tillamook Sweet Cream Unsalted

- 1 lb Macaroni Noodles Elbow

Instructions

1. In an instant pot (ours is a 6qt) add the water, butter, stock, salt, ground mustard, nutmeg and hot sauce.

2. Add the noodles and stir to combine.

3. Close the lid, making sure that the valve is set to seal.

4. Cook on high pressure for 6 minutes.

5. Do a quick release by turning the valve to vent.

6. Open the lid and add the cream cheese along with all of the cheeses.

7. Stir to combine and serve immediately.

Shepherd's Pie Cups

Preparation time

30 minutes

Ingredients

- 1 lb ground beef

- 1/2 Tbs Worcestershire sauce

- 1 tsp salt

- 1 tsp pepper

- 1 tsp dried parsley

- 1/2 cup yellow onion diced fine

- 1 tsp minced garlic

* 1/4 cup butter

* 3 Tbs flour

* 1 1/2 cups beef stock

* 2 Tbs heavy cream

* 12 ounces Peas and Carrots frozen

* Salt and Pepper to taste

* 1 cup shredded cheddar cheese

* 1/2 package McCain® Smiles® Mashed Potato Shapes

Instructions

1. Preheat oven to 425 degrees, and cook 1/2 a package of McCain® Smiles® Mashed Potato Shapes according to package directions.

2.   Leave oven on when finished to finish the shepherd's pie cups.

3. Meanwhile, in a large fry pan, add ground beef, Worcestershire sauce, salt, pepper, and parsley, and cook over medium heat, breaking up beef, and browning.

4. Once beef is browned, drain the grease off it, and remove it from the fry pan into a large bowl. Set aside.

5. In the same fry pan, add onions, and garlic, and sauté over medium heat 3-4 minutes, until onions become translucent, and fragrant.

6. Add onions to the bowl with the browned beef.

7. Add butter to the pan and return to the stove to medium heat, and let it melt.

8. Once melted, use a wire whisk to whisk in the 3 Tbs of flour, forming a paste.

9. Slowly add beef stock, whisking as you add it, until incorporated.

10. It should be thickening nicely as you do this.

11. Once desired thickness is reached (1-2 minutes), add frozen vegetables, heavy cream, and the ground beef and onion mixture.

12. Stir, and heat until veggies are heated through.

13. Taste, and adjust seasoning with salt and pepper as desired.

14. Fill a muffin pan with this ground beef mixture, and top with cheddar cheese, and a cooked McCain® Smiles® Mashed Potato Shape.

15. Put in already heated oven, and cook 4-5 minutes until cheese is melted.

16. Serve and enjoy.

TACO PIZZA

Preparation time

30 minutes

INGREDIENTS

- 2 tubes (8 oz each) refrigerated crescent rolls

- 1 package (8 oz) cream cheese, softened

- 1 cup (8 oz) sour cream

- 1 pound ground beef or ground turkey

- 1-2 envelopes or 2-4 Tbsp taco seasoning, to taste

- 1 medium tomato, chopped

- 2 cups shredded Mexican cheese

- 1 cup shredded lettuce

- optional: avocado, taco sauce, hot sauce, black beans

Instructions

1. Preheat the oven to 375 degrees.

2. Unroll the crescent roll dough and lay out on a large ungreased cookie sheet.

3. Pinch the perforations together to seal.

4. Bake at 375 for 8-10 minutes or until light golden brown.

5. While the crescent rolls are baking, mix the softened cream cheese and sour cream together.

6. Remove any lumps with a whisk. Set aside.

7. Brown the ground beef and drain.

8. Add a can of drained black beans, optional, for more protein if desired.

9. Add the taco seasoning and 1/4 cups of water.

10. Simmer for 3-5 minutes, stirring occasionally.

11. When the crescent roll pizza crust is finished baking, remove from the oven and set aside to cool for 3-5 minutes.

12. Spread the sour cream / cream cheese mixture over the crescent rolls.

13. Sprinkle the ground beef mixture evenly over the top, followed by lettuce, tomatoes, cheese, and any other desired toppings.

14. Cut into serving-size pieces and serve immediately or store in the refrigerator for cold taco pizza to be served later.

Chicken Bacon Ranch Pull Apart Rolls

Preparation time

40 minutes

Ingredients

- 1 15-oz packaged 12-count potato rolls (i.e. Martin's)

- 1 lb thinly sliced deli chicken

- 8 slices bacon cooked and crumbled

- 12 slices colby jack cheese

- ⅓ cup prepared Ranch salad dressing

- ½ cup butter

- 1 Tbsp chopped fresh chives

- 1 tsp garlic salt

- ½ tsp onion powder

- 2 Tbsp grated Parmesan cheese

Instructions

1. Preheat the oven to 350°F. Line a large baking sheet with parchment paper.

2. Using a serrated knife cut through the middle of the potato rolls.

3. Place the bottoms side by side on the pan. Set the tops aside.

4. In a small saucepan over medium heat, melt together the softened butter, chives, garlic salt and onion powder.

5. Brush the bottoms of the sliced rolls with about ⅓ of the seasoned butter.

6. Layer ½ of the cheese on the bottom, then arrange the chicken and bacon crumbles over the cheese.

7. Break cheese slices if needed to fit.

8. Drizzle with Ranch dressing.

9. Top with the final layer of cheese.

10. Brush liberally with butter mixture.

11. Place the tops on the cheese.

12. Brush the remaining seasoned butter on top and sides.

13. Sprinkle with grated Parmesan cheese.

14. Cover loosely with foil. Bake covered for 20 minutes then uncover and bake for an additional 10 minutes or until the tops are lightly golden.

15. Cut apart and serve immediately with additional Ranch dressing, if desired.

Panera Mac & Cheese

Preparation time

30 minutes

Ingredients

- 1 pound medium shells pasta

- 4 Tablespoons butter

- ¼ cup all-purpose flour

- 2 ½ cups milk anything but skim milk

- 4 ounces (about 6 slices) sliced white American cheese from the deli counter, cut into thin strips

- 8 oz extra-sharp white Vermont cheddar shredded

- ½ teaspoon Dijon mustard optional

- 1 teaspoon kosher salt

- ¼ teaspoon hot sauce optional

Instructions

1. Prepare pasta according to package directions.

2. In large saucepan over low heat, melt butter.

3. Whisk in flour and cook 1 minute, whisking constantly.

4. Gradually whisk in milk; cook over medium heat, whisking until mixture thickens and bubbles.

5. Remove from heat.

6. Add cheeses, mustard, salt, and hot sauce, stirring until cheese melts and sauce is smooth.

7. Stir in pasta and cook over medium heat for 1 minute (or until thoroughly heated). Serve immediately.

Pesto Chicken Veggie Meatballs

Preparation time

35 minutes

Ingredients

- 1 pound chicken breast

- 1/2 medium bell pepper, red

- 1 medium carrot

- 1 cup zucchini

- 3 tablespoon pesto

- 1/2 cup bread crumbs, plain

- 1/2 teaspoon salt

- 1 tablespoon olive oil

Instructions

1. Preheat the oven to 375 degrees.

2. Start by preparing the vegetable mixture:

3. Gently pat the zucchini dry with a paper towel or clean dish towel (no need to squeeze all the liquid out of it, just pat off some of the extra moisture).

4. Add to a large bowl with the finely minced carrot and bell pepper.

5. Add in the pesto, bread crumbs, and salt and stir to combine.

6. Fold in the ground chicken breast using your hands or a large fork, and toss together the

chicken and vegetable mixture until it's well-combined.

7. Try not to over-work the mixture.

8. Line a baking sheet with foil or a slipat and drizzle with oil.

9. Using a 1" scoop or a Tablespoon, make small (1-1 1/2") meatballs and place them on the baking sheet. (you can also just use your hands to roll them out)

10. Bake at 375 degrees for 10 minutes.

11. For a bit of browning, broil the meatballs an additional 1-3 minutes. If browning isn't important, continue baking meatballs another 2-3 minutes, or till cooked through.

12. Serve with your favorite sauce, pasta, or on a sandwich. Enjoy!

ALPHABET SOUP

Preparation time

8 hours 15 minutes

INGREDIENTS

- 2-900 ml sodium reduced chicken broth

- 1 lb. cooked chicken

- 1/2 onion, chopped

- 2 stalks celery, chopped

- 2 carrots, chopped

- 1 large garlic clove, minced

- 2 medium bay leaves

- 1 tsp. thyme

- 1/2 tsp. celery seeds

- 1/2 cup uncooked alphabet pasta

- Salt and pepper to taste

- Fresh parsley for garnish

INSTRUCTIONS

1. Add all the ingredients to a slow cooker except the chicken, pasta and salt and pepper.

2. Cook on low for 5-6 hours, won't hurt it if it goes for 8 hours.

3. Half an hour before serving add the chicken and bring back up to a simmer on high.

4. Add the pasta for the last 20 min.

5. Remove the bay leaves and adjust seasoning with salt and pepper.

6. Serve with fresh parsley for garnish.

7. If storing the soup refrigerated, the pasta will absorb a lot of the broth so you may need to add more to serve again this next day.

cauliflower cheese nuggets

Preparation time

22 minutes

INGREDIENTS

- 350g / 12oz cauliflower

- 50g / 1 cup fresh breadcrumbs

- 100g / 1 cup grated cheddar cheese

- 1 medium egg

- 1/4 tsp garlic powder

- 1/2 tsp mixed dried herbs

INSTRUCTIONS

1. Preheat the oven to 200c / 390f and line a baking tray with parchment paper or a silicone non-stick mat.

2. Chop the cauliflower into small pieces and cook it by either boiling or steaming it, which ever is your preference.

3. Once the cauliflower has cooked add it to a food processor and blitz until it has broken down into small pieces.

4. Add the rest of the ingredients and blitz again just enough until they are all combined. You don't want to over-blitz the mixture!

5. Place one large spoon of the mixture at a time onto the baking tray and mould into a round shape.

6. I make about 12 nuggets from this but it will depend on what size you want them to be.

7. Bake in the oven for 12-14 minutes until golden brown.

8. Allow to cool for 5 minutes before serving as this will help them to keep their shape.

9. Serve immediately or store in an airtight container in the fridge for up to 48 hours.

Breaded Chicken Tenders with Buttermilk Ranch Dressing

Preparation time

37 minutes

Ingredients

For the chicken--

- 1/2 cup panko bread crumbs

- 1/2 teaspoon garlic powder

- 1/2 teaspoon onion powder

- 1/4 teaspoon salt

- 1/4 teaspoon freshly ground black pepper

- 1/4 cup grated parmesan cheese

- 4 egg whites or 2 large eggs

- 1 pound chicken breast tenderloins

- 4 teaspoons olive oil

For the Buttermilk Ranch--

- 2 tablespoons mayonnaise

- 2 tablespoons sour cream

- 1/4 cup low fat buttermilk

- 1 tablespoon fresh dill plus 1 teaspoon, finely

chopped

- 1 1/2 teaspoons white wine vinegar

- 1/2 teaspoon garlic powder

- 1/4 teaspoon salt

- 1/4 teaspoon freshly ground black pepper

Instructions

1. Preheat oven to 400 degrees.

2. Set wire cooling rack over a large rimmed baking sheet.

3. Spray rack with nonstick cooking spray and set aside.

4. In a small shallow bowl, whisk together the bread crumbs, garlic powder, onion powder, salt,

pepper and parmesan. In another small bowl, beat the egg whites.

5. Dredge each tender first in the egg whites, then in the bread crumbs, pressing to coat.

6. Put the coated tenders on a plate as you go, repeating the dredging process until all the tenders are coated.

7. In a 12-inch nonstick skillet, heat 2 teaspoons of olive oil over medium high heat.

8. Add ha;f the tenders and cook until golden brown on one side, about 3 minutes.

9. Flip and cook until the second side is golden brown, another 3 minutes more.

10. Transfer to the prepared baking sheet.

11. Add the remaining 2 teaspoons of oil to the pan, and repeat the cooking process with the remaining tenders.

12. Bake until the tenders are golden brown and cooked through, 8-10 minutes.

13. For the ranch dressing, whisk together the mayonnaise, sour cream, buttermilk, dill, vinegar, garlic powder, salt and pepper.

14. Serve the warm chicken tenders with ranch on the side. {My kids used ketchup and BBQ sauce too. Yum yum!}

Queso Chicken Bake Recipe

Preparation time

1 hour 10 minutes

INGREDIENTS

- 3-4 chicken breasts

- 1 can RO*TEL

- 1 can corn, drained

- 1 can black beans, drained and rinsed

- 16 oz Velveeta

INSTRUCTIONS

1. Place the chicken breast in a baking dish flat. Butterfly breasts if they are especially thick.

2. Layer the corn, black beans, and RO*TEL on top of the chicken.

3. Dice the queso cheese into 1/2 inch cubes and spread them evenly over the top of the dish.

4. Cover the dish with foil and bake in a preheated oven at 375F for 45-55 minutes or until the chicken is done and the juices run clear. *if you want the cheese to be a little crispy remove the foil for the last 5 minutes of baking.

5. Remove from oven then remove the chicken breasts from the pan and use a fork or whisk to work the extra cheese into the juices to form more queso sauce.

6. Enjoy! Serve over rice, with chips, or with tortillas

Sloppy Joe Cornbread Casserole

Preparation time

50 minutes

Ingredients

- 15 oz pkg cornbread mix

- 2 eggs beaten

- 1 1/3 cups milk

- 2 lbs lean ground beef

- 1 cup ketchup

- 2 tbsp brown sugar

- 2 tsp yellow mustard

- 1 tsp garlic powder

- 15 oz can corn drained

- 1 1/2 cups shredded cheddar cheese

Instructions

1. In a mixing bowl, whisk the dry cornbread mix, eggs, and milk until smooth.

2. Spray a 9 x 13 baking dish with non stick spray.

3. Spread cornbread batter evenly into dish.

4. Bake at 350 for 20 minutes (cornbread will not be completely baked).

5. Meanwhile, brown and drain the ground beef in a skillet.

6. Mix in ketchup, brown sugar, mustard, and garlic powder.

7. Keep sloppy joe mixture on low heat until cornbread finishing the first baking time.

8. Remove partially baked cornbread from oven.

9. Top evenly with drained corn.

10. Spread sloppy joe mixture evenly over corn.

11. Sprinkle shredded cheese over top of casserole.

12. Return to oven and bake an additional 15 minutes until the cheese is melted and the cornbread is done.

13. Remove from oven and allow casserole to rest 5 minutes before serving.

Sloppy Joes

Preparation time

30 minutes

Ingredients

- 1 Tbsp olive oil

- 3/4 cup chopped yellow onion

- 3/4 cup chopped red bell pepper

- 1 lb lean ground beef*

- 2 garlic cloves, minced (2 tsp)

- 3/4 tsp chili powder

- 3/4 tsp paprika

- 1/2 tsp ground mustard

- Salt and freshly ground black pepper

- 1 (8 oz) can tomato sauce

- 1/2 cup ketchup**

- 1 Tbsp Worcestershire sauce

- 1/2 tsp natural hickory smoke flavor

- 4 hamburger buns

Instructions

1. Heat olive oil in a 12-inch non-stick skillet over medium-high heat.

2. Add onion and bell pepper, saute until nearly tender, about 6 minutes.

3. Scoot to one far side of the pan.

4. Crumble in beef, let sear until browned on bottom, about 2 - 3 minutes.

5. Then turn and start to break up beef and toss with peppers and onions, continue to cook 2 - 3 minutes or until nearly cooked through.

6. Drain fat from beef.

7. Add garlic, chili powder, paprika, mustard and season with salt and pepper to taste and cook beef through, about 1 minute, tossing occasionally.

8. Stir in tomato sauce, ketchup, Worcestershire, smoke flavor.

9. Reduce heat and simmer until heated through, about 2 minutes (thin with a few tablespoons water or broth as needed).

10. Serve warm in hamburger buns.